Travel and Nutrition:

How to Make Healthy Choices

By

Paula I. Birth

Copyright © 2016 by Paula I. Birth

ISBN: 1523669128
ISBN 13: 9781523669127

DEDICATION

This book is dedicated to all those who inspire me on a daily basis. Most and foremost, my loving husband, Brent, who has supported me through the years and all the adventures my path has yielded. His support, interest, and encouragement in my nutritional journey have been unyielding, and for that I say thank you, my love. My granddaughter, who has juvenile arthritis, has been an inspiration for me to research how nutrition can affect conditions of all types, and I will keep looking for ways to help her. Lastly, I also want to mention Colin and Jayne Watson for their encouragement and guidance through this process of writing my first book. You are special people, and I thank you as well.

Table of Contents

INTRODUCTION

Both travel and nutrition can often be challenging. I will give you in this book what has worked for me in not only maintaining my weight but eating healthy. Yes, you can eat out with clients while traveling and maintain nutritional quality. The first and foremost requirement is to be committed to your health and be disciplined in your choices.

First, what is your support system both at home and at work? Let's start with your home or personal support system. It is crucial for a successful nutrition plan to work that the main people in your life understand your reasons for choosing this plan. For me, I have always been health conscious, but when I was diagnosed with a high level of gluten sensitivity and gallbladder disease, nutrition became a focal point. After much trial and error, my family knows that if I don't remain disciplined, the implications and physical effects are not good.

Even my two grandchildren know Nana can't eat the same as they do. Often my granddaughter will ask, "Can you have this, Nana?"

In addition, I share my nutritional values with my coworkers for a couple of reasons. First, if they understand my reasons and needs for the choices I make when eating out, they are more apt to be supportive.

Secondly, by knowing my nutritional values, they'll take them into consideration when ordering out, catering events, or just selecting eating establishments. I truly have an awesome support team both personal and professional.

As a teenager, I struggled with my weight and self-image, tried many of the fad diets, and attended gyms starting around age sixteen. This was back in the mid-seventies when our society wasn't as heavy as it is today, and my generation all wanted to look like one of Charlie's Angels. It wasn't until my first year out of high school that I finally started to see progress from my years of dieting and working out. By early 1980, I had reached a weight and physical image that made me feel good. That year, I married my husband of now thirty-five years, who has been a huge supporter in everything I have done.

For many years, I maintained my weight and was doing well with no issues. Along came the 1990s, and my husband was diagnosed with high triglycerides. So I started doing research on various foods and the impact they have on the body, looking for something to help him lower his triglycerides and cholesterol. (He is not a fan of medication, nor am I. Our perspective is that this is putting more chemicals in our bodies. Now, I grant you, there are times this is the measure one must take, but I like to be more conservative whenever possible.) Through this research I found the Protein Power plan by Michael Eades, MD, and Mary Dan Eades, MD. After in-depth research, we started the program, which is a calculated high-protein, low-carb plan based on your individual body composition. As a result, his triglycerides came down, and yes, I dropped some weight as well.

For many years, this is the plan we followed. Our diet today is still high-protein, low-carb with some modifications, as we are all individually different and our bodies need different things. For my husband, he can maintain at a higher carb level than I, and he has a broader group of carbs that have a neutral effect on him. This was the baseline plan we followed until 2010, when I started to reduce my gluten intake selectively. This was solely based on additional research and the impact I read that gluten and GMOs (genetically modified organisms) can have on our bodies.

All was going well until the fall of 2013, when I had a severe abdominal attack that landed me in the emergency room. Our first thought was my appendix was rupturing, but that was ruled out. I learned I have gallbladder disease; my gallbladder functions only 25 percent of the time. Of course, I was scheduled for surgery at 6:00 a.m. on a Monday. I wasn't feeling good about surgery and wanted to get a second opinion from a holistic doctor, but there wasn't enough time. Well, it so happens that the Sunday night before my surgery, I got a call from the surgeon himself, stating he had a family emergency and must go out of town. He instructed me to call his office in the morning and reschedule. I hung the phone up and was actually happy that the surgery was canceled. In the morning, I called a holistic doctor whom several individuals highly recommended to me, Deborah R. Bernstein, MD, of the Holistic Healing Center, but the doctor's office explained new patients were placed on a waiting list. I explained my situation and asked if there were any way to see me sooner. The receptionist said she would put me on the list to speak to the doctor but noted their appointments were booked for two months. I thanked her and hung up.

I decided I would not call the surgeon to reschedule just yet. On Friday of that same week, I got a call from Dr. Bernstein's office, stating they had a cancelation on Monday and the doctor would move me to the top of the list since I was pending surgery. I said yes, I would be there.

Now, Dr. Bernstein's office is in Lahaska, Pennsylvania, two hours from where I live. After I arrived at her office, Dr. Bernstein spent approximately two hours with me, taking a medical and personal history for as far back as I could remember to my childhood. I had also taken with me the blood-test results, ultrasound, and gallbladder scans that were done for her to review. After several hours of good discussion on my health and nutritional habits, she stated she couldn't promise that my gallbladder wouldn't need removing at some point in time, but she felt she knew the cause of the problem and would like an opportunity to try to correct the issue. I told her I was willing to try and understood the fact that at some point, there may be no avoiding surgery. I then provided her with my food journal of several years. After reviewing it, she said it was good that I had been journaling, and this provided her with good information. She told me she would like me to do an elimination diet and proceeded to provide the instructions of how to do this. Then she would see me in four to six weeks. I left her office feeling confident this would work.

I went through the elimination diet and followed the FODMAP group of foods. (FODMAPs are Fermentable Oligo-Di Monosaccharides and Polyols, or short-chain carbohydrates or sugars.) There is a FODMAP under resources for your reference. It was amazing to see how my body responded. The next-to-last food group I tried was dairy, and I had a small reaction to it. I learned that I tolerate goat products best. The last food group was grains—*bam*! This was the culprit. This indicated I have a high gluten sensitivity. Even though for the past several years I had been selective about not eating gluten, I wasn't avoiding it.

With making lifestyle changes in my nutritional plan of no gluten but still eating high-protein, low-carb, I still have my gallbladder nearly three years later and feel great. I've maintained a good weight, body mass index (BMI), and self-image. Now in addition to avoiding gluten, I also take some natural supplements prescribed by my doctor to assist my digestive system and remove the stress on my gallbladder.

I've managed to do this even while traveling a minimum of 14 days a month as an executive in business development.

However, about a year ago, I was feeling like I was slacking on my program and workouts, so I looked for an online trainer and found Colin F. Watson. In our first session, Colin asked me to keep a food journal. I responded with I do that and have for the past five or six years. He was shocked and asked, "Can you send that to me?" So I e-mailed him my logs.

The next time we met online, he stated, "You don't need me. These journals are great. Do you really eat like this and travel?"

Yes, I told him, but I needed to know someone was holding me accountable for my nutrition and exercise.

We continued to work together, and in one session, he suggested I should do something in this field because I am so passionate and dedicated. I actually had considered going back to school for a nutritional degree, but at age fifty-five, I decided I didn't need all the math. He then encouraged me to look into health coaching and said there were good programs online. I took his advice, researched some schools, and ran them past him until I found the best one for me, and enrolled in the Institute for Integrative Nutrition in New York City, described on its website (http://www.integrativenutrition.com/) as the world's largest nutrition school.

Several sessions later, Colin suggested that due to my success with travel and weight management, I should write a book. Thus, you are reading my story.

Now for the good stuff! I will share with you my philosophies, theories, and practices, as well as what works and what doesn't work for me. These tips also can apply to those of you who don't travel. The only difference is, you don't need to pack! Keep in mind: We are all different, and your individual nutritional needs definitely come into play. Even so, my hope is that you will have at least one takeaway toward better nutrition and health.

Paula

THE PROCESS

When preparing for a trip, whether business or pleasure, I always make sure the accommodations I have booked include a refrigerator and sometimes a kitchenette, depending on the length of stay. I pack enough travel packets of protein powder, Athletic Greens®, Quest Bars (protein bars) or something similar, beet powder, a shaker bottle, and travel scale. In my briefcase and purse, I always have nuts, fruit, and Quest Bars just in case I get hungry. If I have something good, nutritious, and satisfying for a snack, then I am less apt to eat something I shouldn't.

When I arrive at my destination, I locate a natural- or organic food store to purchase water, organic fruits, flax milk, mixed greens, nuts, and goat cheeses. If my stay is for a week or more, I will also purchase egg whites, cut-up veggies, and bacon. Omelets are a favorite of mine in the morning or the evening, if I don't have any dinner plans and I have access to a kitchen. Depending on my schedule of client meetings and events that include meals, I plan my menu accordingly. If at an event a salad might be my only option, I usually have a protein shake before going. Often times the entrées will be breaded or filled with something that is high in carbohydrates and gluten. When others have alcohol, I have a seltzer with lime for several reasons. The first is this is lower in calories, and the second is I keep my wits about me. The last reason is the gluten. Alcohol has a stalling effect on weight loss and can also cause weight gain. A glass of wine or a seltzer with gin or vodka are best to keep the calorie count down. When you start into mixed drinks with fancy names, the calories—mostly from sugar—are high. If you are a beer drinker, you have some lighter options, including gluten-free beer.

One won't have too much of an effect if you feel the need to partake.

Typically, when you're eating out, every menu has something you can have no matter what your nutritional requirements are. The key is to ask questions about the menu. Don't be shy. It's your body, and you deserve to know what is in your food and how it is being prepared. For the most part, eating establishments respect you, and the finer ones will even send the chef to the table to inquire more about your nutritional needs. Those of us with gluten allergies can always fall back on a salad with grilled meat minus the croutons. However, I have noticed over the past year that the number of establishments offering a gluten-free menu is growing. Other restaurants are offering options for other food allergies such as onion or dairy. Many will provide you a listing of the menu and all the ingredients and allergens in various dishes. Once again, the key is asking!

A typical day of travel for me would look something like this: First thing in the morning, I weigh myself. I have a 4-oz. glass of Bragg Organic Apple Cider Vinegar and warm water, or one lemon and warm water. Next, I take my supplements and vitamins with 10 oz. of water and Athletic Greens®. Sometimes I will add 1 T. of organic red-beet powder to my mix. Depending on the time, I either make or order an egg-white omelet filled with green veggies and feta cheese with two or three strips of uncured bacon (this is my preference, as it contains no added nitrates, only those naturally occurring) and some fresh berries. If I am rushed, I will mix a protein powder, usually a Quest travel packet with less than 4 g of net carbs, with 8 oz. of water or unsweetened flax milk (to keep sugar intake low), some ice, and maybe some berries into the blender. If there is no blender, I use a shaker bottle. I use and recommend the following brands of protein powders: Quest, BioTrust, and Athletic Greens®. I've tried many on the market, but these are low in carbs and have a high protein content, as well as taste good. The nutritional content and taste is something you can verify through the label and your experience.

Two to three hours after breakfast, I will have an apple, some raw nuts, or a Quest Bar with a bottle of water or organic oolong tea. Lunch would consist of a mixed-greens salad with 3 to 4 oz. of a lean meat or a pack of tuna (plain or various flavored versions; just read the label for the sugars) and some berries. If I am dining out with clients for lunch, I might choose a white fish, green veggies, a tossed salad, or a 4-oz. steak filet. I tend to eat fish and chicken five out of seven days and salads with protein shakes on the other days.

Once again, two to three hours after lunch, I have a snack similar to the one after breakfast.

Dinner when on the road almost always is broiled or grilled fish or poultry with mixed greens salad and green veggies. Occasionally, I will have a yam or quinoa. Because of my gluten intolerance, I do not have breads or starches, for the most part. Many restaurants are now offering gluten-free breads, so the option is there. However, for me personally, I find that the calorie count is high, and the carbs have a negative effect on me. The other reason for this is I have a low tolerance for carbs. It's all about individuality, and for me, this is how my body responds best. Lastly, it is key to drink a minimum of eight glasses of water a day, as this flushes out fats. I tend to drink between 72 and 100 oz. of water a day in addition to morning coffee and oolong teas throughout the day. The impact of coffee is very individualized; some can tolerate only moderate amounts, and others, such as I, can have an expresso and go to bed. On long travel days, a midday power coffee gives me that extra push and is satisfying. To make a power coffee, add 1/2 tsp. butter and 1 tsp. MCT coconut oil to your 8- or 10-oz. coffee. This can also be done in the morning. Add a scoop of protein mix, giving you a good start with healthy fats and protein.

What is important is that you make the commitment, stay dedicated, and focus on your goals. It's OK to treat yourself occasionally once you reach your goal. In fact, it is good to shock your system about every eight to ten days so the body doesn't become complacent. You can do this in one of two ways. First, if you do low carbs as the norm then a day of cheeseburger and fries and something sweet is good to do. The second option would be to do a good cleanse. Not sure how to cleanse you can contact me at the email provided later in the book, and I will work with you. If you are on medications and under a doctor's care, consult your doctor prior to doing this.

EXERCISE

The key is to move and have accountability. A fitness tracker makes you aware of how much you're moving, especially if you are someone who sits at a desk for work. I have tried various trackers and most recently have been using the Fitbit Charge HR as it monitors and records heart rate, calories, steps, and sleep patterns. This type of tool will allow you to make challenges with others online and is a good motivator. If you can't get out to walk, you can walk in place. Just move the body. Take ten to fifteen minutes in the morning or whenever you can, and do some light resistance training starting with 2- to 5-lb. weights and working up to ten to fifteen pounds of weight for eight to ten reps. This is just for tone and not muscle building. If you haven't been active in a while, this is a good place to start. You want to exercise at a pace where you can have a conversation without feeling breathless. Once you reach that threshold, increase the number of repetitions and continue the process. Try to move ten thousand steps a day, and work up from there. This is the default on most fitness trackers, but don't let this be a deterrent. Start where you are comfortable but challenged and work upward. Progress in small increments will yield lasting results. Once again, if you have medical concerns, consult with your doctor prior to attempting this. It won't take you long to get the process and see the progress. Oh, and remember drink your water.

For those of you who are road warriors, make the best of the layover in the airport and walk the terminals, or take the stairs. Walk to your appointments or dinner. Leave the cab or car service behind whenever that's possible and safe. For me personally, my highest step days are travel days, even with the long flights.

NUTRITION

As I said earlier, we are all different, and your individual nutritional needs play a big role in what works for you in maintaining a healthy weight and lifestyle. The key is to keep a journal to record what you eat and learn how your body reacts to different foods and portions. This is why weighing yourself every morning is important. As you look at your weight and the previous day's food intake, you will begin to learn what your body reacts to, both good and bad. Eating clean, organic, non-GMO foods will also affect your weight, and I do believe that avoiding gluten is good for everyone, not just those with the sensitivity. There are a lot of studies on how GMO foods and gluten have impacted our weight and health as a society.

If you are interested in knowing more about this, and working with me as a health coach to develop a plan, guide you, and hold you accountable, I would love to work with you. My website is www.rebalancewithpaula.com, and my e-mail is paula@rebalancewithpaula.com. It doesn't matter where you are located. We can meet via Skype.

KEEPING A JOURNAL

Journaling is key, as I have mentioned before. It not only keeps you accountable, but it also keeps you aware of your daily intake and allows for you to make good decisions based on daily choices. For example, if I have two eggs over easy, two strips of bacon, and two gluten-free pancakes for breakfast, my nutritional count would be about 413 calories, 19 g of fat, 20 g of protein, and 37 g of net carbs.

I learn midmorning I have a dinner meeting at a fine steak restaurant. Based on my morning intake, I know that for lunch I need to keep my calorie and carb intake low, so I go with a salad and grilled chicken, knowing my dinner will be a steak, most likely a 4- to 6-oz. filet mignon with a green veggie like asparagus. If berries are on the menu, that would be my dessert. If there's no such dessert option, then I might go with brown rice. By journaling, I know throughout the day where I am in my nutritional count.

At first, this might seem time-consuming and a pain, but there are so many good apps today with large databases that can help. In a few short weeks, the few items you eat that might not be in the database are on your device, so this becomes a matter of selection. I have tried several journaling apps, and my preference is MyNetDiary (http://www.mynetdiary.com/). If your preference is to keep a notebook that works too. What matters is not the form of journaling but that you do journal.

On the road, I find that there are more and more natural or organic eating establishments. At the minimum, a lot of your finer places now offer natural or organic options on the menu. As I stated before, don't be afraid to ask to speak to the chef to make changes to meet your needs, and you will maintain or even lose weight on the road. It works! I have been doing this for about six years with much success. In fact, sometimes I return home several pounds lighter than I left.

BALANCE

A key to good body weight is not just watching what you eat but getting a good night's rest, a minimum of eight hours. Also drink plenty of water and exercise even if it is only walking thirty minutes a day. Healthy relationships, which are part of what I call primary food as well as your spiritual and mental well-being. If there is stress in a relationship or any part of your life you will soon be out of balance. Take time to reflect or meditate; know what makes you happy and feel good. When all this is in balance, you will tend to make better eating decisions and will be less likely to eat out of stress.

LOSING THE FAT AND KEEPING IT OFF

Finding a balance between proteins and carbohydrates is the key to losing the fat and keeping it off. For most, the five foods I'll outline below should be eliminated from your pantry and diet, and you will see a change in belly fat, as well as fat in general. These five foods cause us to store fat.

The first is not exactly a food but a drink that my generation grew up thinking was good for us. Concentrated orange juice and concentrated fruit juices are high in sugar. Through the concentrating process, the fiber and nutrients are removed, leaving you with sugar water. This causes your blood sugar to rise, which puts the body into fat-storing mode.

Our blood-sugar levels are directly related to our insulin levels, and insulin is our fat-storing hormone. Sugar is the main culprit here, as it is in processed foods. Excess sugar in our diets in one thing we have too much of. When you read the labels of processed food, you most likely see one or more of the following: high-fructose corn syrup, dextran, dextrose, and fruit-juice concentrate. All of these are just fancy names for sugar, causing the same impact on your insulin levels.

The second food to remove is margarine, as it is loaded with trans fats, which affect your good and bad cholesterol. In order to give it a longer shelf life, margarine contains hydrogen, which has a negative effect on our HDL (or "good" cholesterol) and boosts our LDL (or "bad" cholesterol). It also causes plaque to build on our arteries. Instead of margarine, eat butter. Butter has fat also, but it is a saturated fat that our body burns as fuel.

Third on the list is whole-wheat breads and high-carb comfort foods. Once again, these cause the insulin levels to spike, and the body goes into fat-storing mode. The key is to balance carbs with proteins.

Number four on the list is processed soy such as soy milk, tofu, and soy protein. During processing, this food is stripped of good nutrients.

Lastly, number five is corn. I don't mean any corn, but genetically modified corn that was developed initially to fatten livestock.

The key to all of this goes beyond these five foods, and that is to read labels. Hopefully, these five will open your eyes enough to make you want to read labels and understand the content of what you are putting in your body. If you would like to learn more on this subject, I suggest looking at the US Food and Drug Administration's website (http://www.fda.gov/), as well as googling the subject.

WHERE TO START

So, where to start? Pack healthy snack options, and at the minimum in the beginning, give up starches and push away when you've had enough to eat. Just because there is still food in front of you doesn't mean you have to eat it. Ask for a box, and take it with you. Reduce the amount of intake you normally have, move more, drink more water, and you will start to see changes.

If you don't travel, these same principles apply. You just don't have to pack.

In 2010, the President's Cancer Panel issued a report recommending when consumers should buy organic produce and when this is unnecessary (http://www.pbs.org/wnet/need-toknow/health/the-dirty-dozen-and-clean-15-of-produce/616/). The group put together two lists, "The Dirty Dozen" and "The Clean 15," compiled using data from the US Department of Agriculture on the amount of pesticide residue found in nonorganic fruits and vegetables after they had been washed. When conventionally grown, the "Dirty Dozen" fruits and vegetables tested positive for at least forty-seven different chemicals, with some testing positive for as many as sixty-seven, according to the report.

"The Dirty Dozen" list includes:

- celery

- peaches

- strawberries

- apples

- domestic blueberries

- nectarines

- sweet bell peppers

- spinach, kale, and collard greens

- cherries

- potatoes

- imported grapes

- lettuce

All the produce on "The Clean 15" bore little to no traces of pesticides, the report states. This list includes:

- onions
- avocados
- sweet corn
- pineapples
- mango
- sweet peas
- asparagus
- kiwifruit
- cabbage
- eggplant
- cantaloupe
- watermelon
- grapefruit
- sweet potatoes
- sweet onions

At the minimum, buy organic to avoid the dirty dozen. I do this on the road, and when home, this is a normal practice. I understand switching to organic can be more expensive than non-organic so do this at the very least. I like to think that if one spends money on good quality food it is less likely they will need prescription medications.

Next, try to eat lean meats and fish (sashimi is a favorite) two or three days a week. I recommend a good lean steak or red meat from grass-fed animals once a week. Some of you will need to have red meat more often. The portion size should be four to six ounces raw, about the size of your palm when cooked. If the portion is too large when eating out, it is OK to take some with you. Just ask for a takeout box. Don't feel like you have to finish everything on your plate.

Green veggies are the best when trying to drop the pounds, as they are lower in starch content. A salad of mixed greens with cucumber, tomatoes, onion, peppers, and 1 oz. of cheese is good fiber and is filling. I would suggest oil and vinegar as dressing until the pounds begin to drop. Most salad dressings are loaded with gluten, sugar, and lots of high-calorie fillers.

For starches, think outside the box and try grains like buckwheat, quinoa, brown rice, and others. Most menus at the minimum will offer brown rice or sweet potatoes. It is important to give the body good carbs for energy. Carbohydrates provide your body with the glucose it needs to function properly. Two types of carbohydrates exist: complex carbohydrates and simple carbohydrates. Complex carbohydrates take time to break down into glucose. Foods rich in complex carbohydrates and fiber are called good carbohydrates. Simple carbohydrates include sugars found in foods such as fruits and milk products and sugars added during food processing. Foods rich in white flour and added sugars are called bad carbohydrates. Something to remember when eating grains is that our primal ancestors used carbohydrates as an elective energy source, and their primary source was protein. The eating of grains is a result of modernization. The key is getting the mix right, which goes back to keeping a journal.

Dessert is not forbidden. Just look for low-sugar items such as fruit, berries, sugar-free JELL-O, and light pudding. Watch out for chemical sweeteners, such as the ones in colored packets. Try to use stevia, Truvia®, honey, or natural raw sugar.

Snacks are good. Just try to have things like Quest Bars, Atkins bars, raw veggies, beef jerky, or nuts. Those who love sweets can make a bowl of Quest ice cream at night. Mix a scoop or two of flavored Quest protein powder, a cup or more of crushed ice, and a cup of unsweetened flax or coconut milk in your blender for a great protein snack before bed. Studies have shown that when looking for a snack before bed, you should focus on protein. Foods high in protein will not only make you feel more full and satisfied; they'll also boost your metabolism and burn more calories while they digest. That means you'll be burning fat while you sleep! Another good snack that helps burn body fat at night is cherries. An abundance of supportive data on lean proteins, fruits, and veggies, as well as the superfoods and their impact as good before-bed snacks, exists. If you would like more details on this, I suggest you google the subject.

Coffee or tea, especially oolong, is good in moderate amounts. The same goes for all I have mentioned. Enjoy in moderation, and treat yourself every once in a while. It will do your body good.

SUPPLEMENTS

This is an area where I would say to do some of your own research and then speak to your doctor. However, that said, just like our food, supplements often have fillers, so be sure to read the labels and purchase a natural product. It is usually good to take a natural vitamin, but once again, here I would recommend deferring to your doctor.

NAVIGATING MENUS AND EATING ESTABLISHMENTS

The key to keeping a norm during travel is in menu navigation. Ask for water with lemon first, and sip on it as you look over the menu. Read the ingredients, and ask how things are prepared, even for breakfast. You will be surprised at the added ingredients that a server might tell you. The hidden items are usually a lot of sodium, starch, or bad fats. These are the three items that will contribute most to weight gain when eating out. Ask for sauces on the side, minimal oil in cooking, and broiling the meat, if possible. Asking for your meat prepared naked is a good way to communicate no seasonings or added sauces. Avoid breading and items marinated in a sauce, especially if purchased that way from a food supplier and not prepared from scratch by the chef. Most fine establishments use virgin olive oil or coconut oil, which is good. However, there are still some chain restaurants using lower-grade oils, which are not good for you. So ask and be aware. Grilled veggies are great as long as the oil is minimal. Instead of french fries or starch, I will ask for a vegetable, tossed salad, or fruit. And I pass on the breadbasket, even if it is gluten free. If you are avoiding gluten, ask if the food is prepared in a non-contaminated area. If the food is gluten free but the area isn't, you could have problems. Kitchens that are truly gluten free use separate pans, utensils, and grill surfaces.

Next is portion size. Your meat serving should be the size of your palm. If larger than that, ask for a take-out box and remove the remainder before starting; you will be less tempted. If the restaurant has a small-plates menu, look it over as these tend to contain the portion size we should be eating as a society. When the server comes for your order, remember to ask questions. If they won't substitute something, tell them to leave it off your plate. While waiting for your meal, have another glass of water and relax.

If you are gluten sensitive, many restaurants now offer gluten free menus and gluten-free options. However, it's extremely important to be very careful and very clear when you order gluten-free food at a restaurant. While it is possible to have great gluten-free meals without incident, you must be very specific to avoid any mishaps in food preparation or cross-contamination.

Some tips to remember. Look for restaurants certified by the Gluten-Free Restaurant Awareness Program (GFRAP), operated by the Gluten Intolerance Group of North America (https://www.gluten.org/). About 1,600 independently owned restaurants in the United States, Canada, and

Germany have been GFRAP-certified as safe for gluten-free guests.

Restaurants are listed on the GFRAP website, http://www.glutenfreerestaurants.org, by location and style of food. The National Foundation for Celiac Awareness offers Gluten-Free Resource Education and Awareness Training (GREAT) to equip chefs, restaurants, and cafeterias with the knowledge and tools to safely provide customers with gluten-free meal options. For more information, visit http://www.beyondceliac.org/kitchens/.

Look also at websites from individual restaurants and restaurant chains to see whether they post gluten-free menus. Some establishments, especially chains, list specific ingredients and allergen information online.

When ordering from a gluten-free menu, inform the restaurant staff about the severity of your celiac disease and the need to prepare food without any cross-contamination.

Select a few favorite restaurants and develop a relationship over time. Chefs at small, local places know the menu and can help you select items that are safe. If you eat at a chain restaurant, choose one that offers a gluten-free menu. Be aware that chain restaurants often use prepackaged dishes, which might mean that the kitchen staff has little control or knowledge of specific ingredients.

INTERNATIONAL TRAVEL

This is more complicated, especially with a food allergy, and requires strictly applying all of the previously mentioned tricks and habits. When traveling in foreign countries, the most important thing is asking questions about the menu. If you do not speak or read the language of a particular country, have someone write in its native language what you are allergic to before your trip. Prior to traveling to China and Hong Kong, I asked a colleague write down what I couldn't eat and what my allergy consisted of so that I could show this to servers abroad. Most often, there was someone abroad who spoke both languages that could interpret for me.

When uncertain, stay with safe foods like grilled chicken, seafood, green veggies, and fruit. In China, I often ate from street vendors as I could pick the meat and veggies and watch as they were prepared and cooked on open fire.

Traveling in Europe is somewhat easier. I found that if I took a gluten block, some of the grains didn't bother me. Recently there has been several articles written on this topic and it is one I plan to explore further.

SAMPLE MENUS

In the chapter titled "The Process," I discuss how I eat when traveling. Here are some sample menus.

Day 1

Breakfast

Apple cider vinegar or water with lemon

Athletic Greens

2 eggs

3 slices Applegate bacon (find where to buy at http://www.applegate.com/)

1 slice low-carb bread, such as Nature's Harvest (optional)

Fruit such as 24 raspberries or 1/2 cup strawberries or blueberries

8 oz. water

Coffee or tea

Snack (two to three hours after breakfast): choose one with 8 oz. water

1 medium-size apple with 1 T. peanut butter

Quest Bar

24 almonds natural unsalted

1/2 cup unshelled pistachios unsalted

Berries measured as above with a Quest Protein Powder shake one scoop

1 (1 1/2 oz.) bag Quest Protein Chips

Lunch

Pouch of tuna with or without low-carb wrap

2 cups lettuce

½ cup mixture of sliced onion, broccoli, peppers, and 1 oz. light cheese (as salad dressing, use 1 T. each oil and vinegar, as much as you need)

Fruit of your choice as listed above

Snack (two to three hours after lunch): choose from above options with 8 oz. water

Dinner

4 oz. skinless chicken breast, broiled or sautéed with 1/2 tsp. coconut oil

1/2 cup green veggie of your choice (not peas)

1/2 sweet potato done in microwave with some butter, if you like

A choice of fruit from above

8 oz. water

Snack (two hours after dinner): choose one from below with 8 oz. water

Shake made with Quest Protein Powder one scoop

Quest Bar

2 oz. cheese

1/2 cup cottage cheese and 2 oz. Applegate lunch meat

3 oz. of grilled chicken

Day 2

Breakfast

Apple cider vinegar or water with lemon

Athletic Greens

Omelet made with 2 eggs and 4 oz. egg whites, stuffed with green veggies and 1 oz. cheese

3 slices Applegate bacon

Fruit: choose 24 raspberries, or 1/2 cup strawberries or blueberries

8 oz. water

Coffee or tea

Snack (two to three hours after breakfast): choose one from Day 1's daytime options

Lunch

3 to 4 oz. grilled chicken or shrimp on salad described below 2 cups lettuce

½ cup mixture of sliced onion, broccoli, peppers, and 1 oz. light cheese (as salad dressing, use 1 T. each oil and vinegar, as much as you need)

Fruit choice from breakfast options

Snack (two to three hours after lunch): choose one from Day 1's daytime options with 8 oz. water

Dinner

4 to 6 oz. steak or lamb, broiled or grilled

1/2 cup green veggie of your choice (not peas)

1/2 cup quinoa or gluten-free pasta

Fruit choice from breakfast options

8 oz. water

Snack (two hours after dinner): your choice of one from Day 1's evening options with 8 oz. water

Day 3

Breakfast

Apple cider vinegar or water with lemon

Athletic Greens

1 cup oatmeal

6 oz. egg whites scrambled with ¼ veggies and 1 oz. cheese

8 oz. water

Coffee or tea

Snack (two to three hours after breakfast): choose one from Day 1's daytime options with 8 oz. water

Lunch

Quest Protein Powder shake one scoop

Fruit choice from Day 1's breakfast options

Snack (two to three hours after lunch): choose one from Day 1's daytime options with 8 oz. water

Dinner

4 oz. skinless chicken breast, broiled or sautéed with 1/2 tsp. coconut oil

1/2 cup green veggie of your choice (not peas)

1/2 sweet potato done in microwave with some butter, if you like

Fruit choice from Day 1's breakfast options

8 oz. water

Snack (two hours after dinner): choose one from Day 1's evening options with 8 oz. water

Day 4

Breakfast

Apple cider vinegar or water with lemon

Athletic Greens

2 eggs

3 slices Applegate bacon

1 slice low-carb bread such as Nature's Harvest (optional)

Fruit: choose 24 raspberries, or 1/2 cup strawberries or blueberries

8 oz. water

Coffee or tea

Snack (two to three hours after breakfast): choose one from Day 1's daytime options with 8 oz. water

Lunch

Pouch of tuna with or without low-carb wrap

2 cups lettuce

Mixture of sliced onion, broccoli, peppers, and 1 oz. light cheese (as salad dressing, use 1 T. each oil and vinegar, as much as you need)

Fruit choice from breakfast options

Snack (two to three hours after lunch): choose one from Day 1's daytime options with 8 oz. water

Dinner

4 oz. skinless chicken breast, broiled or sautéed with 1/2 tsp. coconut oil

1/2 cup green veggie of your choice (not peas)

1/2 sweet potato done in microwave with some butter, if you like

Fruit choice from breakfast options

8 oz. water

Snack (two hours after dinner): choose one from Day 1's evening options with 8 oz. water

Day 5

Breakfast

Apple cider vinegar or water with lemon

Athletic Greens

2 eggs

3 slices Applegate bacon

1 slice low-carb bread, such as Nature's Harvest (optional)

Fruit: choose 24 raspberries, or 1/2 cup strawberries or blueberries

8 oz. water

Coffee or tea

Snack (two to three hours after breakfast): choose one from Day 1's daytime options with8 oz. water

Lunch

2 to 3 hardboiled eggs

2 cups lettuce

½ cup mixture of sliced onion, broccoli, peppers, and 1 oz. light cheese (as salad dressing, use 1 T. each oil and vinegar, as much as you need)

Fruit choice from breakfast options

Snack (two to three hours after lunch): choose one from Day 1's daytime options with 8 oz. water

Dinner

4 to 6 oz. fish of your choice, broiled or sautéed with 1/2 tsp. coconut oil

1/2 cup green veggie of your choice (not peas)

1/2 sweet potatoes done in microwave with some butter, if you like

Fruit choice from breakfast options

8 oz. water

Snack (two hours after dinner): choose from Day 1's evening options with 8 oz. water

BAKING AND COOKING WITH FEWER CALORIES

Do you like to bake? Learn to use sugar substitutes that measure one for one to sugar like Swerve or Monk Fruit. The taste is great, and the calories are much less. Try alternative flours like buckwheat, almond, and coconut. Even if you don't need to be gluten free, explore the taste and texture of these other options.

Here are some of my favorite recipes for snacks, sweets, and entrées. I would like to hear your thoughts once you have tried not only the recipes but any of the suggestions, concepts, or ideas provided in this book. Please e-mail me at paula@rebalancewithpaula.com.

Low-Carb Pumpkin Muffins

Found on various sites: http://www.jarilove.com/, http://www.victoriawellness.com/, http://5050fitnessnutrition.com/, and http://www.tristanknellfitness.com/

Here's a muffin that isn't sugary, starchy, and devoid of nutrients— like the muffins at your favorite coffee shop. These muffins are rich in beta-carotene and contain half an egg's worth of high-quality protein. The delicately sweet flavor will satisfy and have you coming back for more.

Ingredients

1/2 cup coconut flour (find at natural-foods store)
2 teaspoons ground cinnamon
1/2 tsp. ground nutmeg
1/4 tsp. ground cloves
1/2 tsp. baking soda
1/2 tsp. salt
1/2 cup canned pureed pumpkin
6 eggs
3 T. coconut oil, melted
1/3 cup honey
1 tsp. vanilla extract
12 pecans for topping

1. Preheat oven to 400 degrees Fahrenheit. Oil muffin pans.

2. In a medium bowl, combine the coconut flour, spices, baking soda, and salt.

3. In another bowl, add the pumpkin, then add the eggs one at a time,

mixing well after each addition. Add coconut oil, honey, and vanilla.

Mix until well combined.

4. Add the flour mixture to the pumpkin mixture; blend with a whisk until

most lumps have disappeared.

Spoon into prepared muffin pan, filling each muffin two-thirds full.

Bake for 18 to 20 minutes or until golden.

5. Place on wire rack to cool. Top each muffin with a pecan. Makes

12 servings

 Per serving: 127 calories, 7 g fat, 230 mg sodium, 11.7 g carbohydrates, 3 g fiber, and 5 g protein.

Crock-Pot Refined Sugar-Free, Dairy-Free Fudge

Author: Brenda Bennett of the blog Sugar-Free Mom
(http://www.sugarfreemom.com/) Prep time: 5 min.

Cook time: 3 hours

Total time: 3 hours 5 min.

Ingredients

2 1/2 cups sugar-free chocolate chips* (See Note)
1/3 cup coconut milk
2 tsp. liquid stevia or 1/4 cup raw honey
Dash of salt
1 tsp. pure vanilla extract

1. Stir chocolate chips, coconut milk, stevia (or honey), salt, and vanilla in a small 3- or 4-quart Crock-Pot. Cover and cook on low 2 hours.

2. Uncover, turn off, and let sit (no stirring, please) for 1 more hour.

3. Stir well for 5 to 10 minutes, until smooth.

4. Line a 1-quart casserole dish with <u>parchment paper,</u> and pour in mixture. Cover and refrigerate 3 or 4 hours until firm.

5. Unmold onto cutting board. Slice into ½ inch chunks. Makes 30 servings.

Nutritional Information: Per serving: 78 calories, 5.8 g fat, 3.7 g saturated fat, 10.9 g carbohydrates, 0.1 g sugar, 1 mg sodium, 2.7 g fiber, 1.4 g protein.

Notes : * If you can't find sugar-free or grain-sweetened chocolate chips, Enjoy Life is an allergy friendly brand. You also can use chocolate chips that have the highest percentage of cocoa in them.

SNACKS

Choose any:

1/2 banana, sliced
1 kiwi, sliced
1/4 cup strawberries, sliced
2 tsp. chia seeds
1 to 2 cups cut celery, carrots, and cucumbers
1 cup mixed berries (blueberries, strawberries, raspberries, and blackberries)
1 medium apple, sliced and dipped into 1 T. peanut butter

SMOOTHIES
Author: Isabel De Los Rios, author of *Beyond Diet: Stop Counting Calories, Start Eating Well and Start Living*

Berry Spinach Smoothie
2 cups spinach
1/2 cup blueberries
1/2 cup strawberries
1 cup coconut milk
1/2 cup ice
2 tsp. chia seeds

Mix in blender until smooth.

Berry Smoothie
1 cup blueberries
1 cup raspberries
1 cup coconut milk
2 tsp. chia seeds

Blend until smooth.

Quest Protein Powder Smoothie

1 scoop favorite flavor of Quest Protein Powder
1 cup crushed ice
1 cup unsweetened flax milk

Blend till milkshake smooth.
(Note: To make ice cream, add more ice and blend till the texture of ice cream.)

Be creative, add any fresh fruit and or veggies to any of these suggested smoothies. Explore the various forms of milk like, flax, almond, cashew, cocoanut and many others to create your own smoothie recipe. Have fun, enjoy healthy eating.

ENTRÉES

Baked Chicken with Roasted Veggies

Author: Isabel De Los Rios, author of *Beyond Diet: Stop Counting Calories, Start Eating Well and Start Living*

Ingredients

1 (4 to 5 oz.) chicken breast
1/4 cup mushrooms
1/2 zucchini, sliced
1 yellow squash, sliced
1 tsp. olive oil or coconut oil
Salt and pepper to taste
1 tsp. dried oregano
2 cloves garlic, minced, divided

Preheat oven to 350 degrees Fahrenheit. Line a baking sheet with

aluminum foil. Arrange vegetables on sheet and drizzle with oil.

Sprinkle with salt, pepper, oregano, and half of the minced garlic.

Place chicken in an oven-safe baking dish. Brush on olive oil. Sprinkle with

salt and pepper and remaining garlic. Cook all for 30 minutes.

No-Bean Turkey Chili

Author: Isabel De Los Rios

Ingredients

1 tsp. coconut oil

1 carrot, diced
1 celery stalk, diced
1 T. tomato paste
8 oz. ground turkey
1 tsp. chili powder
1 tsp. cumin
1 clove garlic, minced
2 cups diced tomatoes
2 cups chicken broth

Heat coconut oil in Dutch oven over medium heat. Sauté all vegetables until soft, about 10 minutes. Stir in tomato paste. Add turkey and cook all the way through, stirring constantly. Add spices, tomatoes, and chicken broth. Stir. Bring to a boil, and boil until chicken broth is mostly cooked off, about 20 minutes. Makes 2 servings.

Veggie Omelet

Ingredients

2 eggs or 4 oz. egg whites
Salt and pepper to taste
2 T. cilantro, chopped
1 small tomato, chopped
1 T. red onion, chopped
4 mini sweet peppers
1 oz. feta cheese

Coat a skillet lightly with coconut oil. Heat whisked eggs in skillet over medium heat until the sides begin to form; add remaining ingredients except the feta cheese. Add the cheese once the omelet has started to form; cover with a lid for 1 minute. Remove lid and fold omelet; flip once and serve.

GLUTEN-FREE PANCAKES

Author: Minimalist Baker Prep time:

15 min.

Cook time: 10 min.

Total time: 25 min.

Ingredients

1 cup brown rice flour
3/4 cup white rice flour
1 cup gluten-free oat flour

1 cup buckwheat flour (ground from raw buckwheat groats)

1/4 cup yellow cornmeal
3/4 tsp. xanthan gum
1 tsp. salt
1 T. baking powder
1/2 T. baking soda
1/4 cup granulated sugar
1 egg
1 to 1 1/2 cups low-fat buttermilk or nondairy milk
1 T. melted butter or coconut oil

1.   Add all dry ingredients in a bowl, and whisk or sift until well combined. Reserve 1 cup of dry mix; store the remainder for another use.

2.   To make pancakes, whisk together egg, buttermilk, and butter or coconut oil. Add reserved cup of dry mix. Batter should stream out of a measuring cup, not glop. If batter appears too thick, add another egg or more buttermilk for proper texture. Let batter rest for 5 to 10 minutes.

3.   Preheat griddle to medium heat. Lightly grease surface; add 1/4 cup of batter for each pancake. Cook for 3 to 4 minutes per side, or until bubbles form on top and the edges appear dry, checking around the 2-minute mark to ensure they aren't too brown. Adjust heat as needed. Flip pancake.

4.   Cook for 1 to 3 minutes more, or until the other side is brown and the pancake feels firm when lightly pressed with a spatula. Serve with butter and honey or syrup. Yields about 10 pancakes.

Note: Store leftovers in the freezer. To reheat, simply thaw for 30 seconds in the microwave and then toast in a toaster until warmed through.

CONCLUSION

As I write this, it is two and a half years since I was diagnosed with gallbladder disease. I recently had the same diagnostic tests run, which showed my gallbladder is now functioning 56 percent of the time, up from 25 percent. I did this with just nutritional lifestyle changes and natural supplements called LVGB and HCL by Designs for Health to ease the digestion process. In addition, my weight has stayed within a five-pound range. Most important, I feel great. My hope for you is that what I have shared will benefit you or someone you know in some way.

Foods suitable on a low-fodmap diet

fruit	vegetables	grain foods	milk products	other
fruit banana, blueberry, boysenberry, canteloupe, cranberry, durian, grape, grapefruit, honeydew melon, kiwifruit, lemon, lime, mandarin, orange, passionfruit, pawpaw, raspberry, rhubarb, rockmelon, star anise, strawberry, tangelo Note: if fruit is dried, eat in small quantities	**vegetables** alfalfa, bamboo shoots, bean shoots, bok choy, carrot, celery, choko, choy sum, endive, ginger, green beans, lettuce, olives, parsnip, potato, pumpkin, red capsicum (bell pepper), silver beet, spinach, squash, swede, sweet potato, taro, tomato, turnip, yam, zucchini **herbs** basil, chili, coriander, ginger, lemongrass, marjoram, mint, oregano, parsley, rosemary, thyme	**cereals** gluten-free bread or cereal products **bread** 100% spelt bread **rice** **oats** **polenta** **other** arrowroot, millet, psyllium, quinoa, sorghum, tapioca	**milk** lactose-free milk*, oat milk*, rice milk*, soy milk* *check for additives **cheeses** hard cheeses, and brie and camembert **yoghurt** lactose-free varieties **ice-cream** substitutes gelati, sorbet **butter substitutes** olive oil	**tofu** **sweeteners** sugar* (sucrose), glucose, artificial sweeteners not ending in '-ol' **honey substitutes** golden syrup*, maple syrup*, molasses, treacle *small quantities

Figure 1

RECOMMENDED SITES

Quest products:

www.quest.com

Protein Power plan:

www.proteinpower.com

BioTrust:

http://rebalancewithpaula.biotrust.com/shop.asp

Athletic Greens:

www.athleticgreens.com

Colin F. Watson, personal trainer:

www.colinfwatson.com

Deborah Bernstein, MD:

www.drbholisticmd.com

Isabel De Los Rios, author of *Beyond Diet: Stop Counting Calories, Start Eating Well and Start Living*

www.beyonddiet.com